The POWER Of YOGA
With Adriana of Yogado

The POWER of YOGA
© Adriana Silva
www.yogado.com.au

All rights reserved. No part of this publication may be reproduced, stored in a retrieval system, or transmitted in any form or by any means, electronic, mechanical, photocopying, recording or otherwise, without the prior written permission of the author.

National Library of Australia Cataloguing-in-Publication entry

Author: Silva, Adriana, author.

Title: The POWER of YOGA / Adriana Silva.

ISBN: 9780992538606 (paperback)

Subjects: Hatha yoga--Handbooks, manuals, etc.

Dewey Number: 613.7046

Published with the assistance by www.inhousepublishing.com.au

Preface

I write this book not only to tell the story of my yoga journey, but also to encourage all who pick it up to "have a go" and see what yoga can bring into their lives; whether it be for a physical, emotional or spiritual reason, irrelevant of race, age, sex, religion or beliefs. This book The POWER of YOGA is a brief insight into the benefits of yoga.

Having being brought up in the East and now living in the West since 1975, I am fortunate to have had the influence of both worlds, respecting all cultures and religions; all have paths leading to the pinnacle of the mountain.

My yoga journey started in 1977 and I am still on this journey today, sowing seeds. I encourage you to start today, just for ten minutes, and let your life be changed, tapping into contentment, happiness and peace within yourself.

I have written this book in a very simple form. I love reading down-to-earth, simple books and I hope all who pick this book up will find at least one little crop of knowledge that they can harvest and reap.

My life is always guided by these words of Matt.7:12: "All things whatsoever ye would that men should do unto you, do ye even so to them."

I also try to live by the standards of the great Mahatma MK Gandhi: "It is claimed that realisation of God in the heart makes it impossible for an impure or idle thought to cross the mind."

Acknowledgements

I am thankful to all whose paths I have crossed during my journey, and for the wisdom that I have gained from them.

I am thankful to all persons on my yoga journey, and especially to all my students who have taught me at each class. I apologise if I have ever been intolerant or not as compassionate as I should have been.

I thank the authors, too many to name, whose books I have enjoyed and which have taken me to amazing places.

This book was put to seed over 15 years ago, and is still being watered with all my learning experiences. I have published only parts of these experiences as there is possibly too much information to share all at once. My next book is already in the "hot house", growing, ready for harvest next season!

Important note: The information in this book is not a substitute for medical care. Please seek medical advice before beginning any exercise routine.

CONTENT

Part 1
    My Journey Into Yoga   1
    Yoga History   7
    Breathing Practise/Pranayama with   10
    Sleep Enhancement

Part 2
    Breast Cancer   19
    Multiple Sclerosis   22

Part 3
    Practical Yoga for Busy People   27
    Workplace Yoga   34
    Chair Yoga (Also for Special Needs   37
    and Nursing Homes)
    Meditations Seated   41
    Self-healing   46

Part 4
    Kids' Yoga   49
    Games for Kids   57
    Relaxation for Kids   61

Part 5
    Yoga Dictionary   69
    Reflection   71
    Final Thought   73

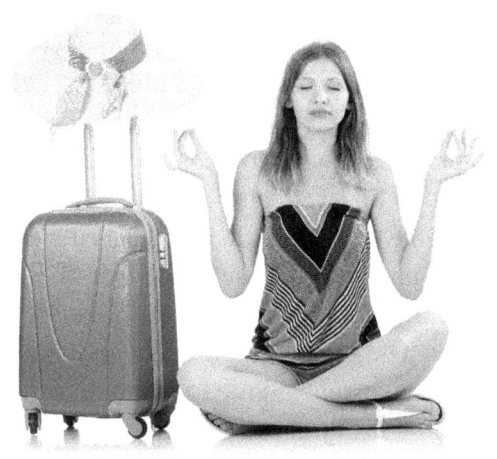

Part 1

My Journey Into Yoga

I have always been a bookworm. I remember from the age of six "reading" the Sunday Times paper with dad in his arm-chair. I would follow his eyes and hold the paper for him. As I grew older, dad and I would share the paper. I would read my part of the paper spread on the floor as it was too big to hold in my little hands. As I grew older, I kept reading more and more books, which have given me wisdom along life's journey. My father encouraged me, and I have finally been able to put thought and action into words!

My yoga "seed" was planted in 1977 when I was invited to a yoga class. I knew from the first class that this seed needed cultivation. Over the years, through getting married and having a family, my seed was not nourished properly, but I always watered it twice a day through practise. I went for classes every week and also to workshops and retreats. I travelled to India, doing yoga every day with an Indian yoga guru. Some of those workshops and retreats were facilitated by dedicated teachers from all over the world from who I drew much knowledge. The hundreds of books and magazines that I have read have enabled me to reap the fruits of yoga. I still feel my journey ahead has much more to offer.

Most of the time when I was practising yoga, my eldest son Johann was training to be a personal trainer. He would join me and comment on my dedication to the art and ask why was I not sharing it with others. On his insistence that my expertise would benefit the future gym he intended having, I decided to finally put all my dedication and yoga journey into a piece of paper, graduating through the International Yoga Teachers' Association. This was a very thorough course in comparison to all the other courses I researched. In 1977 during my first few classes, I remember doing the poses in a very aerobic style, trying to achieve a flat tummy and all the benefits to make myself "body beautiful", not realising the greater inner beauty to be unearthed.

What is a yoga practise?

Yoga is the conscious unfolding of oneself whereby physical, mental and spiritual nature is moulded into perfection, to enjoy total wellbeing, just how we were created and meant to be.

We should all be living happily and at peace, and to get to this we need to free ourselves of physical and emotional burdens and worry. In our modern society we tend to live by stringent planning. Planning is necessary to "keep the clock working" on time. Sometimes we cannot keep up with this clock and that's when bodies crumble and there is a price to pay, mentally and physically. Yoga helps you to live happily one day at a time, in the present moment, accepting all that is negative and positive, and knowing that the negatives can become positives with yoga practise.

The human body is made up of the union of the soul (jivatman) or "inner voice/the spirit/the ego" and the universe (paramatman). A healthy body is required to live a happy, fulfilling life. If our bodies are weak, sick and not strong, we cannot enjoy a fruitful life.

A healthy body and a strong mind will enable us to experience the kingdom of God within us, where we all can live in complete harmony with each other. I liken this to our bodies. No matter how small a part of the body is injured - for example, if we break our toe - it affects and imbalances our whole body. Similarly, graduating to the bigger picture, from individual, family, friends, country, world, universe ... it is the same principle.

To attain a peaceful, balanced mind and body we need a proper diet and exercise.

Our body is comprised of many parts; muscles, cells and blood vessels, to name a few. To be conscious, we need movement through our muscles. Active muscles are healthy muscles. If our muscles or tissues are not exercised and stretched, we stoop and become hunched, and the muscles will ultimately lose their correct function. When our muscles, cells and blood vessels are not working properly, our body is not in balance - our muscular, circulatory, respiratory, digestive and elimination processes are not functioning properly, and we are more prone to "dis-ease". In our present society, this is affecting all of us in one way or another. In yoga asanas/postures, we stretch, flex, contract and strengthen our fascia, ligaments and muscles with breathing (this will be explained in detail in our next chapter).

Nature provides protection, food and movement to all living beings. In the Stone Age there was little security or effective weapons. It was all manmade simplicities and fleeing to save oneself, whether a bird, animal or human being. To be able to flee, strength in movement was needed. This was through the constant use of limbs and muscles. In this modern age we do not use our limbs or muscles the way we should and as a result there is a chain reaction; physically, mentally and emotionally, resulting in dis-ease of our bodies when we are not in tune with nature.

The yoga asanas/postures help the body, both externally and internally, to be healthy. The wonderful aspect is coordinating the breath (inhalation) with the stretching; then the pause in the breath before the exhalation, giving a chance to feel the muscles, the extent of the stretch, whether the stretch can be taken further, the posture, and generally making any adjustments, and being fully aware of how the body is, and what is happening to it. Then, on the exhalation, going deeper into the posture and moulding into the posture without any unease. After all this, the tension is removed and you are gradually being taken to a state of softening and thus feeling more alive and full of energy!

Who can do yoga?

I asked this question the first time I attended a class. Yoga is for everyone. As long as you can breathe and are alive, there is some form of yoga that can be done. Yoga does not have to be physical. It works on the body, mind and spirit. If the physical part is not for you, try the breathing, meditating or relaxation.

My body is like a tree,
Reaching for the sun.
Turning my leaves
Lest I shall not gleam.
As I grow older
I grow from within.
Nurturing myself
Lest I shall not be.
My branches spread out,
My leaves give shade,
My trunk for children
What a journey I have made!

**Om Shanthi, Om Shanthi
(peace to the universe)**

Yoga History

Yoga is the oldest science and art of self-development in which the body, mind and spirit unite for better health, internally and externally. Yoga originated from India over five thousand years ago. The word "yoga" means "union" in Sanskrit, an ancient language from India.

"Yoga is a way of life". The asanas/postures mould the body like a potter. Once the shape is moulded it is fired with the heat of breath, then touched with the brush of a mandala and etched with the silence of Om. All converging into beauty from within, with love for the wondrous beauty of perfection.

The Ten Commandments are there to put us on the straight and narrow. Similarly the eight limbs of Classical Yoga.

Eightfold Path of Yoga; Eight Limbs of Patanjali

Yama:	Avoidance – personal and social behaviour
Niyama:	Observance of inner discipline and re sponsibility
Asana:	Discipline of physical body
Prana:	Force or energy (breath control)
Pratyahara:	Withdrawal of senses inwardly
Dharanaya:	Concentration; focusing of mind
Dhyana:	Uninterrupted meditation without object
Samadhi:	Absolute bliss (devotion, meditation and contemplation)

Hatha Yoga is covered by the first five limbs of the eightfold path. Raja yoga (inner) is the last three limbs.

I endeavour to follow the first five limbs through regular practise and discipline. I often wondered at my early yoga classes why relaxation is necessary at the start of a class, not realising that this was to quieten the mind and prepare the body inwardly. It also made me realise that our mind and body need to be in synchronicity to reap fruitful results.

Posture

Ideally a comfortable seated position is a good posture to ground the body at the base of the spine, keeping the spine erect and tummy tucked in, chin slightly down towards the chest to lengthen the neck. Hands in a comfortable position. Always imagine with eyes closed that the body in this position is in the shape of a triangle, starting at the apex, the head. Many classes however start off in a lying-down position due to the time of day. This is okay as long as one doesn't drift off to sleep. Consciously relax the muscles and mind and take awareness inward, away from worldly distractions.

If we have a strong spine and abdomen muscles, all our organs will be in place and this will benefit the wellbeing of our body. By keeping the spine stretched and supple, it can support the body in any posture, as well as the nervous system. The abdominal cavity contains the internal organs, i.e. the stomach, intestines, liver and spleen. Good, healthy, strong muscles and proper functioning of the organs helps in the digestive and eliminative process and also promotes a fit, toned and healthy body. The other parts of our body, our limbs, the upper and lower back, the neck and head extend from the spine and abdomen. If our spine and abdomen muscles are strong our whole body will also be.

When tension attacks, it attacks in various places. The most frequent areas are the shoulders and neck, and sometimes the buttocks. The asanas/postures illustrated in this book will help to reduce this tension and gradually you will be able to avoid letting little things whirlwind into bigger things.

This saying tells it all: **"I am more accepting than expecting!"**

Breathing Practise
(Pranayama)

What is pranayama? In Sanskrit, Pran means "oxygen" and Ayama means "to extend and control". The action of inhaling, exhaling and controlling our breath is pranayama. Breath is our life force. If there is no breath there is no life. It is as simple as that. When we are in a state of panic or fear we breathe fast and shallow. When we breathe slowly, steadily and deeply we are in natural control of ourselves. Watch a baby or toddler breathe while resting, deep into the belly, not into the upper chest.

When we are in control of our breath, all the five elements of the body (fire, water, air, ether and earth – the tattwas) are in harmony.

To explain this concept further: there are seven main chakras/energy centres along our spine. The five elements correspond with the first five chakras.

Earth: Our connection to earth, being grounded and absorbing the scents around us, being nourished and nurtured. Centred at the end of the spine in line with Muladhara is the first chakra (red).

Water: Our body is 80% water (on average), we cry, sweat and excrete fluids. Centred along the spine at Swadhisthana (just above the first chakra) is the second chakra (orange).

Fire: The heat within us on all levels in mind and body, our expressions and reactions. Centred along the spine at the navel area, Manipura is the third chakra (yellow).

Air: Our connection to this world through our breath, our touch sensations. Centred along the spine in line with the heart, Anahata is the fourth chakra (green).

Ether: Our connections, in all forms of communication, awareness through vibrations, mantras, sounds. Centred along the spine in line with our throat, Vishuddhi is the fifth chakra (blue)

The five elements relate only to the first five chakras above. There are two other main chakras:
- In between the eyebrows, Ajna (colour purple).
- On top of the crown, Sahasrara (colour pink or white).

All living things on this earth, whether they are in the form of water, trees, animals, stones or plants, breathe. For growth, breath is vital. If there is no breath/air, there is no life. We can live without food for a long time and without water for a shorter time, but without air for a few minutes - death.

Pranayama can help to keep away colds and diseases as a result of the strengthening of the lungs. Pranayama is a sport in itself, very much an active sport, where you can reach a level of increased energy. If done properly, one will actually perspire and can run out of breath. This is good for the body as it removes impurities. Imagine these impurities in our body and not released. Compare the idea to other eliminations like faeces and urine - what would we feel?

What is the correct way to breathe?

When we inhale we breathe air in through the nose, our windpipe and then into our lungs. Usually we always remember to breathe in through the nose. Sometimes when we are eating we get choked. The reason for this choking is because a little air accidentally enters our mouth and it goes to the windpipe with particles of food. The windpipe can only accept air. Another reason we should breathe through our nose is because when the air enters the nose it is warmed when it contacts the mucous membrane. Also there is filtering of dust in the nasal cavity. When you breathe in through the mouth there is no warming or protection of the air, and this can lead to inflammation and diseases of the respiratory system. The lungs consist of numerous cells. These cells absorb air and then separate oxygen from the air and toss out by exhalation the excessive air. The air that is absorbed by the cells in the lung is then sent to the heart for purification of the blood. Deep Yoga breathing and the holding of our breath magnifies this process by strengthening the lungs and the whole of the respiratory system. Shallow or superficial breathing slowly disables the function of the cells in the lungs and this can lead to lung diseases and eventual collapse of the lungs.

Some of the benefits of proper breathing are

- relaxes, to reduce stress and fatigue
- increases lung capacity
- conscious breathing helps to lift energy levels; concentration and mental functions are improved
- oxygenates the blood to cells and increases blood flow to brain

- helps blood to flow properly
- alleviates stress and anxiety
- calms the nervous system

When we breathe in:

- we take air that is warmed to the respiratory system
- the oxygen that is in this air is absorbed by the blood vessels
- the pollutants, like carbon monoxide and nitrogen, are released when we exhale

Pranayama is divided into 3 parts:

(I)   Poorak/inhalation
(ii) Kumbhak/retention of breath
(iii) Rechak/exhalation

Try these exercises:

- Inhale, hold the breath for as long as possible.

- Exhale with full force. Relax tummy and lungs, avoid breath coming in; when comfortable inhale slowly.

- Inhale only taking breath to navel until comfortable; then take breath from navel to heart and then to throat; when you feel you cannot breathe anymore, keep this breath inside you for as long as possible and slowly exhale from navel, heart and throat.

The ultimate aim is to breathe in different ratios, taking small steps first, eg.

Inhale	Hold	Exhale (in seconds)
4	4	4
4	8	4
4	8	20
4	16	20

What we are trying to achieve is, while holding that breath within us, to feel the inhaled air reach all different parts of our body, energising and revitalising us through the flow of fresh oxygenated blood.

Exercise I

Stand tall with arms beside you. Inhale a full breath and hold. Spread both hands in front parallel to the chest. Bend elbows, place fingers on shoulders. Contract arm muscles tightly, hands coming into fists and closed. Exert pressure on muscles, still retaining breath. With closed fists straighten elbows and back to shoulders again. Form lips as if to whistle and exhale all air from lips in a hissing sound until all air is exhaled. At the same time, bring down the arms slowly. Repeat.

This exercise is good for memory, blood circulation and strengthening of arms, chest, back and shoulders.

Exercise II

If you feel tired, inhale through nostrils strongly, retain and then exhale through lips in the form of whistling intermittently, till all the breath is expelled.

Insomnia/Sleeplessness

Causes of people having difficulty sleeping (insomnia) are usually:
- shift workers' variations
- time zones when travelling
- stress
- mental disorders
- physical/emotional pain
- mature persons

Several types of medications are effective for treating insomnia. However, long-term use is not recommended. Many doctors do not recommend relying on sleeping pills for long-term use. It is also important to identify and treat medical conditions that may be contributing to insomnia, such as mental disorders, chronic pain or breathing problems.

Yoga and relaxation provides long-lasting results. How this works is to reduce the temperature of blood flowing to the brain to slow the metabolic rate of the brain to reduce sleeplessness.

Avoid:
- Watching television
- Reading exciting or dramatic books

Ways to improve sleep quality are:
- Listening to soft music
- Using lavender essential oil
- Reading to children
- Massaging soles of feet and calves
- Breathing techniques such as alternate nostril breathing/nadi sodana
- Specific yoga postures
- Listening to a relaxation tape

Alternate Nostril Breathing/Nadi Sodana

Imagine there is a little dim light in one nostril. Close the other nostril. Breathe in and out of the open nostril and every time you breathe in the light gets brighter and it travels along your nostrils to the space between your eyebrows. Close that nostril and open the other nostril and do the same.

Working with both nostrils, fingertips of index and third fingers are placed between eyebrows. Close right nostril with thumb. Breathe in through left nostril up to eyebrows, close left nostril with ring finger, exhale down right nostril. Breathe in through right nostril up to eyebrows, close right nostril with thumb, breathe out through left nostril. This is one full round. Do a few rounds. Imagine a light in between your eyebrows as you breathe in and out. If you are lying down and doing this, preferably lie on your right side.

Be Happy!
Feel Happy!
Live Happy!
Happiness radiates from within.

Peace of mind
Peace of heart
Peace radiates from within

Love you and me
Love is all we need!

Notes

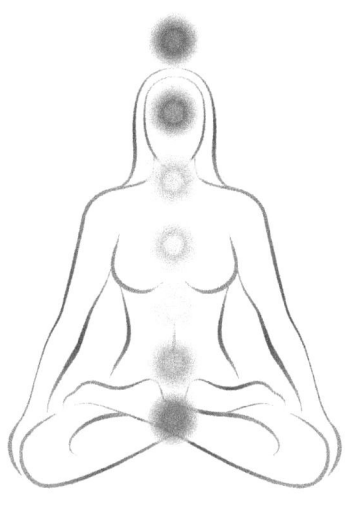

Part 2
Breast Cancer

On life's journey, we all are faced with challenges and a major challenge was in 2003, when I was diagnosed with breast cancer. It hit me like a Tsunami, battering body, mind and spirit.

Breast cancer was the last thing on my mind. I was energetic, youthful, had never smoked or indulged in alcohol. I had also never been for a mammogram. On my doctor's insistence I went for a test, and one month later I was undergoing double surgery.

Unlike Multiple Sclerosis, there were no symptoms. I was healthy and eating a balanced diet. The only factor I can put it down to is stress and my way of dealing with tests and trials, whether it be family, work, financial or simply by being over-sensitive.

When I received the diagnosis, my partner was overseas at his mother's funeral. I was with our three young children. I didn't break the news to the kids or my family until my partner returned home two weeks later. We then decided to do all we could medically to rectify this health issue.

My faith, family, and yoga, helped me on a gentler healing journey, and my recuperation process after surgery was only a couple of weeks. I remember not being able to even lift my left arm where lymphatic nodes were taken out for testing, and then later, it was extremely painful to lift my arm above the shoulder. My yoga training then came into service.

The ward I was in had a full length mirror. I looked at myself in the mirror each day, and using my yoga training:

- I got the straightened arm to move up a centimetre in front
- I got the straightened arm to move up a centimetre sideways a
- I bent the elbow, with fingers on my shoulder, and did the same exercise in front and sideways

My surgeon was very impressed. After a week I was able to take the arm all the way up with my fingers pointing towards the ceiling. As a result of doing specific yoga exercises, I was able to drain away any problem fluid in my arm, and was able to go about my daily duties normally. *(this is demonstrated in website www.yogado.com.au)*

Taking "one day at a time", when I was hit by this "Tsunami", was the best "medicine". There was really nothing I, or anyone else could do. Simply, I did what had to be done medically, and left the rest to the divine. This is my "mantra".

I believe challenges are put before us for a reason. To share my experience with you is one good reason. Since then I have become a better and stronger person by not allowing small things to take over my life, and taking one day at a time.

My next book will give a more detailed insight into my cancer journey and how I coped with it.

Multiple Sclerosis
(MS)

This chapter is dedicated for a number of reasons, but most of all at the request of a friend to any person who is suffering from MS, keen to do yoga, but can find no literature on "Yoga for MS". There are immense benefits from the simple yoga exercises explained in this chapter, as well as on the website ***www.yogado.com.au.***

I have been fortunate to get first-hand experience from a close friend who is facing this challenge, yet living a normal life by being aware of what is happening, taking preventative measures and living happily with the support of her family.

Multiple sclerosis (MS) is a disease in which the body's immune system eats away at the protective sheath (myelin) that covers your nerves. Myelin can be compared to the insulation on electrical wires. When myelin is damaged, the messages that travel along that nerve may be slowed or blocked. Damage to myelin causes interference in the communication between the brain, spinal cord and other areas of the body. This condition may result in deterioration of the nerves themselves, a process that's not reversible.

Yoga is a strategy to use along with oral and injectable medication and muscle relaxants. The yogic stretching and strengthening together with the relaxation and meditation will provide benefit, and make it much easier to perform daily tasks. The balancing postures in yoga can be very helpful to sufferers from MS to help focus, and thus prevent falls.

The symptoms of MS are:

- Visual disturbances, which includes blurred vision, color distortions, loss of vision and eye pain
- Limb weakness and numbness, loss of coordination and balance
- Muscle spasms, fatigue numbness, prickling pain
- Loss of sensation, speech impediment, tremors or dizziness and in the extreme, vertigo
- Bladder and bowel problems
- Mental changes including impaired focusing, attention deficit, memory loss
- Depression
- Paranoia
- Uncontrollable laughter and weeping
- Reflexes, very sensitive in some cases

Symptoms vary widely, depending on the amount of damage and the nerves that are affected. People with severe cases of multiple sclerosis may lose the ability to walk or speak clearly. Multiple sclerosis can be difficult to diagnose in the early stages because symptoms often come and go — sometimes disappearing for months.

The cause of multiple sclerosis is unknown.

Fatigue is a common symptom of multiple sclerosis. Get plenty of rest.

Regular exercise, such as walking, swimming, weight training and other physical activity, may offer some benefits if you have mild to moderate MS.

Some Benefits of Yoga:

- **To improve strength:** A sequence of yoga postures such as Salute to the Sun will increase strength
- **Muscle tone:** Kneeling, sitting and standing postures are very beneficial
- **Balance and coordination:** All balancing and coordination exercises, whether standing or seated, will assist
- **Bladder and bowel control:** Breathing techniques such as pelvic floor breathing will help greatly
- **Fatigue and depression:** The breathing exercises, relaxation and meditation will reduce these
- **Cool down to prevent MS symptoms:** Use cooling-down breath technique (sitali)

Eat a balanced diet. Eating a healthy, balanced diet can help you maintain:

- a healthy weight
- a strong immune system

By practising the strengthening yoga postures good bone health is maintained.

Stress may trigger or worsen MS symptoms. Try to find ways to relax such as:

- yoga relaxation and meditation
- full yoga breathing with background relaxing music.*(as demonstrated in website www.yogado.com.au).*

Notes

Notes

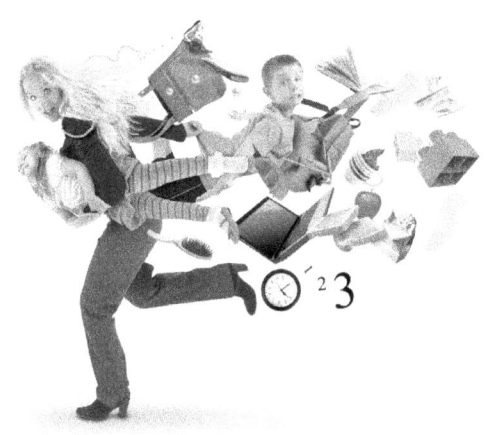

Part 3

Practical Yoga for Busy People

We all lead very hectic lifestyles and sometimes it is hard to find fifteen to thirty minutes for a yoga session at home. Most of us can afford only one or two yoga classes a week, and find it hard to make the time for ourselves, due to home/family commitments. This segment is especially for all those yogis.

In our busy world, it is hard to find the time, to enjoy the stretching, breathing, strengthening and relaxation of the total body. It is all rush, rush!

Whilst in Bed (Cradle Yoga)

I remember as a child, my mother would remark, if anyone was in a bad mood during the day, about "getting out of the wrong side of the bed", had a lot to do with this feeling. When I think about this it does mean something. If I get out of bed in pain or with a negative attitude or thought, my day is not very pleasant. I try to get out with positive feelings, allowing these to unfold throughout the day, like a domino effect.

Doing a few stretches in bed can help this (provided you do not disturb others. I am sure that could put a damper on the rest of the day!).

Stretching front, back and sides of body:

- take a deep breath in, taking arms overhead, stretch the whole body
- point toes towards face and away
- exhale to bring hands beside body
- take left hand up, stretch, then stretch right leg, flexing the toes
- do the same to the other side

We tend to curl in and sleep, and sometimes one side is not aligned with the other. To rectify this:

- lie on your side with hand under your head
- bend top leg at knee and bring knee forward
- tuck tail bone
- hold tummy in

- stretch from the top of your fingers to your toes
- repeat with the bottom leg bent

This stretches the whole side. Remember to tuck the tail and hold the tummy as that holds the hips in place.

Massaging back, neck and spine:

- take both knees to chest
- embrace both legs tightly
- move them from side to side to massage back
- place a hand on each bent knee
- take knees apart, wider than hips
- make circles clockwise and anti-clockwise
- knees bent
- feet flat
- take one knee to chest
- holding leg firmly onto chest to flatten out spine
- if no problems with neck or shoulders, take nose to knee

Working into tummy muscles:

- bend knees
- feet flat
- hands on thighs, breathe in and bring head up to breathe out. Doing this a couple of times
- take opposite bent knee to opposite elbow
- fingers touching back of neck/head

- gently lifting head (if no neck/shoulder problems), and gently coming down onto your back.

This is a mini workout for everyone and anyone, and the wonderful thing is that your body is supported and moulded beneath you, not causing any strain.

Pelvic Floor Breathing:

- take both arms overhead, palms together (or leave arms beside you if you have shoulder problems)
- bend knees with feet flat on bed, hip width apart
- breathe in, exhale tighten pelvic floor muscles and scoop them up towards the navel and at the same time stretching the upper body
- exhale again to keep scooping them up and at the same time, take the navel towards spine. Let go. A few more repetitions

Brushing Teeth:

- take feet wider than hips
- feet pointing out
- tuck tail under
- bend knees in a frog/chair position to strengthen those legs, tummy and back
- lean your back against something to make it easier

At Kitchen Bench:

- holding bench with both hands outstretched
- legs at 90 degrees, feet flat
- bend knees if uncomfortable
- take one leg away as high as possible
- swing that through, toes touching bench floor, foot flat
- knee bent, trying to keep the back foot heel towards the floor to work into those legs, hips and tummy
- Bring feet together in same posture as you started, stretching the spine, pushing the buttocks away
- same with other leg

On Steps/Stairs:

Downward Dog: (higher stairs or steps make it easier especially if you have pains in your joints or high blood pressure. This is working on your whole body, strengthening your arms and legs and at the same time stretching the spine and working into your core).

From **Downward Dog** come into **Upward Dog** working on opening your chest, and it is a counteraction to work into the muscles evenly.

Table top on stairs:

- holding onto the upper stair with hands behind you whilst sitting on a lower stair
- feet hip width apart
- opening chest

- bring shoulder blades close together
- face parallel to floor
- breathe in, tighten the buttocks and lift the body, straightening the arms and exhale
- keep breathing in and out whilst in this position
- This is a much easier version with less strain and the stair will support you to sit down if you feel tired or any discomfort

Side of Bed:

Stand two feet away from bed, feet and hands hip width apart (if experiencing shoulder problems, bent elbows on bed). Push the buttocks away from the bed and shift the weight onto legs. Shift weight onto hands and come forward. Do this a few times to stretch the spine, arms and legs and strengthen the whole body. Hold the navel towards the spine to engage the lower abdominals. This will help with bowel movement as well.

Talking on the phone standing:

Tadasana/Mountain Pose:
- standing tall
- feet hip width apart
- shoulder blades coming together
- opening the chest
- tucking tail and tightening buttocks
- hips opening
- holding core and engaging the abdominals
- chin parallel to floor
- looking straight ahead
- arms hanging loosely beside the body (or

- holding phone with one arm)
- breathe in through feet along spine to stretch body
- exhale down spine through feet
- each time stretching the body with the breath
- standing tall like a mountain

Vrikrasana/Tree Pose
- standing tall
- feet hip width apart
- shoulder blades coming together
- opening the chest
- tucking tail and tightening buttocks
- hips opening
- holding core and engaging the abdominals
- chin parallel to floor
- looking straight ahead
- bring all weight onto one leg and standing tall
- bring other heel to balancing ankle bone
- palms in prayer at chest (if on phone, one hand at chest)
- breathe in through feet, legs, hand/s and start extending arms while breathing in
- exhale and bring hand/s down to chest.

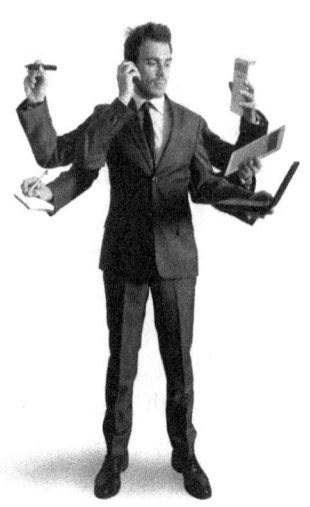

WORKPLACE YOGA

Sitting at a computer or desk the whole day affects your eyes, face, shoulders and back, which will in turn affect the rest of the body. Most of our day is spent at our work place. In order not to be affected by this syndrome of stiffness, rigidity and discomfort, try some of these exercises at your desk.

Sit up straight, feet evenly on floor, steady chair, buttocks evenly on chair.

Hands and Arms
- Bring your palms together at your heart centre, with a bit of resistance against each other, your elbows bent.
- Take the palms out, still together in front of you, elbows straightened
- Separate the arms, palms facing in, facing up, down and to the side, to rotate the wrist. Do this a few times.

- Take arms to the side, bring palms to chest.
- Stretch both arms straight out in front of you with relaxed hands. Make fists and rotate both hands at the wrists around in a circle (clockwise) five times and then anti-clockwise. Repeat.
- Do the same movement above, this time with the arms in line with the shoulders.

Shoulders, Neck and Spine:
- Palms on thighs very loose, roll your shoulders up towards your ears, roll back and let go. Now try it with the breath. Breathe in, lifting shoulders, take it back, exhale and let the shoulders go with a sigh.
- Take left shoulder towards bent left ear, allow right arm to hang gently, fingers pointing towards floor and moving fingers. Same to other side.
- Take arms behind, clasp fingers and open chest, bring chin to chest, take chin up, chin down and gently to left, centre and to right. Lift head, look straight ahead at computer, let go of arms and bring them in front to clasp palms again and work neck as described above.
- Bring elbows together in front of chest, stretch arms out, bend head, take chin to chest and place your fingers at the back of your head; encourage your chin to come down to chest, to stretch the neck and spine. Gently lift head, open bent elbows, take in line with shoulders,

sitting up straight. Take palms together overhead and stretch arms. Take a breath in, exhale, sigh out, bring arms beside, relax, just letting go. Shrug shoulders in one direction, then the other.

Eyes

- Have a sticky note marked with a big dot at the centre of your computer. Focus on this dot (don't move head, only eyes), then:
    - look over the top of the computer
    - return gaze to dot at computer
    - look below computer
    - return gaze to dot at computer
    - look to left side
    - return gaze to dot at computer
    - look to right side
    - return gaze to dot at computer
    - look to top right hand corner
    - return gaze to dot at computer
    - look to top left hand corner
    - return gaze to dot at computer
    - look to tip of nose, using fingertips as focus
    - return gaze to dot at computer

Close your eyes, rub both palms together till you generate heat and place palms on your eyes to rest and massage.

This is a wonderful therapeutic exercise. Ideally should be done when your eyes are tired or two to three times a day whilst at office.

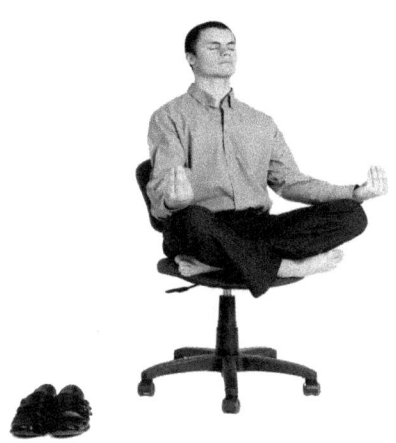

Chair Yoga
(Also for Special Needs and Nursing Homes)

As we age our body often limits us from rising off a mat, or kneeling/sitting on the floor. Chair yoga is a modified version to make it more practical and gentler, using a chair as your prop.

The advantage is that your feet are flat on the floor to ground yourself, and your buttocks are on the chair, thereby stabilising the upper body, especially the spine, whilst in a seated position.

A good example of this is the Spinal Twist *(see website www.yogado.com.au).* I personally find this posture stronger than on the mat, especially when you lift one leg over the other; to really stretch into those hamstrings and relieve discomfort from sciatica. Holding the back of the chair with the twist really opens the chest to maximum, and squeezes the waist, to get those internal organs flushing.

In the standing positions use the wall as a prop, eg. Tree and Dancer.

I recently had an advanced student compare a mat and chair yoga class. She found the poses on the chair quite strenuous, and more opening and releasing.

As we age, our bones get weaker and thinner, increasing frailty and risk of fracture. Hatha Yoga, with its weightbearing postures combined with the breathing, prevents osteoporosis.

What is Osteoporosis?
It is a disease of the bones that leads to an increased risk of breakage as a result of the bones deteriorating and altering bone mineral density.

The form of osteoporosis most common in women after menopause is referred to as Primary Type 1 or Postmenopausal Osteoporosis. Primary Type 2 usually occurs after age 75 and can be seen in both females and males. Type 2 can also happen at any age to both genders as a result of chronic medical problems, disease or even prolonged use of medications (eg. steroids).

The postures in yoga, especially the weightbearing ones, while applying pressure, example, Downward Dog, helps the bones to thicken and become stronger and helps retention of calcium. *(see website www.yogado.com.au for a complete class with relaxation/meditation)*

While watching TV, if you are short of time and feeling sluggish, would be an ideal time to put some of the chair yoga exercises to practise. As one student said, "while

I am watching the kettle boil, I do some stretches at the sink".

Another good time is while travelling, whether in a plane, car, truck, practically anywhere, as long as there is leg and stretch room. Keeping the blood flowing will also prevent deep vein thrombosis which is very common on long journeys.

Wheelchair and special-needs persons find chair yoga challenging, yet at the same time therapeutic, as the stiff muscles and joints are specifically targeted. Muscles and joints are slowly worked, getting movement again in a gentle stress-free way. The small steps achieved bring a grin and confidence to their faces. To witness this is a joy.

The gentle bending, stretching and moving of yoga quietly works into muscles and balance, and improving coordination. Over a period of time, with continued practice, the basic yoga stretches become easier, and the mind is quietened, focused and relaxed.

My mum is presently in a nursing home where I have volunteered to teach yoga classes. Many of the residents participate and find it very beneficial. The exercises are very gentle, and all are done seated. They try their best to move their hands and legs, ankles and wrists. They love the breathing, the focusing on a candle, relaxation and last but not least, the benefits of self-healing.

I have noticed some of them some of them at the start of the class, with shaky limbs; some cannot place their feet flat on the floor. By the end of the class there are no shakes and the feet are evenly flat, and they are amazed at the transformation.

Getting positive feedback at the end of a class and seeing smiles on their faces brings me joy. That's when it feels good to have given something to the community.

Meditations – Seated

- coming into a comfortable seated position
- feet flat on the floor evenly
- arms hanging loosely, fingers pointing towards floor
- take a deep breath in through your nose as you lift your shoulders, exhale through the mouth with a loud sigh. As you exhale letting go of any chattering monkey thoughts or pain, whether it be emotional or physical. Do that once more.
- take your chin to chest gently
- breathe in and look gently up
- exhale through your nose to bring your chin down
- again in your own time
- leave your chin on your chest
- gently walk the chin along the chest to the right
- take another breath in and exhale to centre
- inhale, gently walk the chin to the left
- take another breath in, and exhale to centre
- lift your head gently as you breathe in
- exhale and turn to the right
- breathe in, exhale and turn to the centre
- same on other side
- breathe in and lift right shoulder towards your ear and encourage the ear towards your shoulder
- exhale and let go of ear and shoulder

- same on other side
- take both your shoulders towards your ears with a deep breath in
- exhale and sigh it out go the shoulders. Do that once more in your own time. Breathe in again and at the same time lifting head and stretching it towards the ceiling, exhale and let go of shoulders. Do this again, trying to keep the shoulders relaxed. How do you feel so far?

If your arms are hanging loose bring them onto your lap in a comfortable position.

Visualisations
(There are 3 different visualisations to follow)

1.   Take your awareness to the base of your spine. Imagine your spine as a tube, and at the base of your spine two little golden marbles. Now breathe in to bring the marbles up along your spine in line with your shoulders, exhale through your nose and take each marble along each arm to your palm. Breathe in and take the marbles back to the top of the spine in line with your shoulders. Exhale down to the base of your spine. Breathe in for the count of four, your whole upper body is completely relaxed. Keep the two marbles at the base of your spine, breathe in and exhale each marble along your legs to your feet. Breathe in and bring the marbles to the base of your spine. Breathe in for the count of four. How do your legs feel, begin to feel no endings to your feet, they are becoming one with the floor. Your lower body is completely relaxed. Gently breathing in and out of your nose, watch the cool air touch your nostrils as you breathe in, and as you breathe out, watch the warm air

touch your nostrils. Stay in this calmness for as long as you wish, just watching that breath. You are the captain of your ship!

2.   Imagine a rectangle, of any size, at your forehead. Breathe in along the short side, exhale along the long side; breathe in short side, exhale long side. Keep going along this rectangle. With each exhalation feel the body letting go and relaxing. Now imagine a golden light at the middle of your rectangle in between your eyebrows. Take your awareness to this light and gently focus on it. On each exhalation imagine this light spreading to fill the rectangle and gradually filling your head, neck, shoulder, arms, chest, buttocks, tummy, legs and feet, completely filled with this light. The light is seeping out through your skin to form an aura around you. Feel your body becoming light and now a floating sensation. Feel yourself swirling in space with all the other stars.

Bring your chin to chest and look straight ahead, left shoulder to ear, exhale and let go. Same movement to the other side. Take a deep breath in and lift both shoulders, exhale and let go of any residual negativity or pain. Stretch both legs wide, take a deep breath and take both arms overhead, widen and stretch the whole body, flexing the feet. Place both palms on lap, looking straight ahead. Reflect on how you are feeling. Stay with this calmness.

3.   Breathe in deeply, into your feet and legs, tense, tense, tense and let go the breath through the mouth.
- Breathe into your buttocks, tense, and let go.
- Breathe into your arms, make fists with your hands, tense, exhale and let go.

- Breathe into your shoulders, take them up and back, tense, and let go.
- Breathe into your face, make a prune face, stick your tongue out, raise your eyebrows, tense and let go.
- Now breathe in deeply through your feet, legs, buttocks, chest, arms, shoulders, face, tense the whole body rigid like a stick, exhale, and let go.

Feeling a sense of release and calmness within. Are there any thoughts still lingering, watch them, and let them go along that conveyor belt.

Watching and feeling the cool breath as you breathe in, and as you exhale feel the warm air touching your nostrils. As you breathe in watch the chest and shoulders rise and as you exhale watch them descend.

- Bring your chin to chest
- chin to right along chest
- back to centre
- to opposite side
- lift head
- take right shoulder towards ear
- let go
- take left shoulder to ear
- let go
- take a deep breath in and lift both shoulders
- exhale and drop shoulders heavily to let go of any residual negativity or pain
- stretch each leg
- take a deep breath and take both arms overhead, palms together

- stretch the whole body
- place both palms on lap
- reflect on how you are feeling

Self Healing

- Take your awareness to your navel. Imagine a blue healing light at your navel. Inhale into this blue light, exhale and take it to your upper body, filling your whole upper body with this blue healing light

- Breathe into your navel again, the blue light, exhale and send it into your lower body, completely filling your lower body

If there is any part in your body that needs healing, imagine that area as being grey. Breathe into the blue light, exhale and send it to this grey area. Imagine each grey cell turning blue, healing and re-vitalising that area. The whole painful area turning blue while you massage it with your breath.

If you are experiencing any emotional situation, breathe into the blue light and as you exhale, sending that situation away, out of your mind, out of your body, to the universe. Allow the universe to deal with the situation.

If there is anyone who needs healing, physical or emotional, send the blue light to that person/s.

Notes

Notes

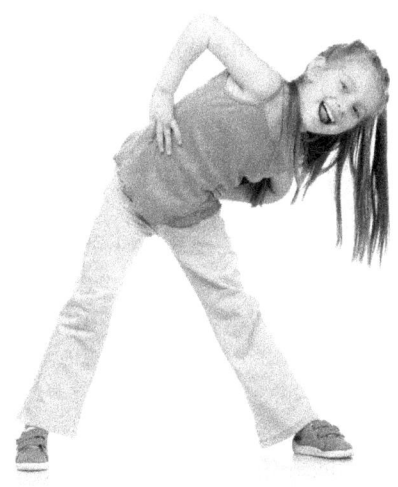

Part 4

Kids Yoga

As adults we are so serious. As children we simply live for the moment, doing all that is needed for that moment and not carrying negatives and mental luggage to the next day.

Pets never hold grudges and lighten us up in the dreariest of times. Your pet dog did something wrong and he was chastised in the morning. However when you come home after work your dog is always there to greet you. Sometimes I wish I could reach this level of enlightenment! This is how we are meant to live, for the day, in peace and happiness.

Kids are the same, their memory span is a positive thing, in that negatives are erased so quickly.

I enjoy teaching kids yoga, relaxation and meditation. I find myself becoming one with them, and temporarily erasing all the worries of the world. Most kids have a lot of inbuilt energy and this has to be channelled to get them into a correct frame of mind.

A yoga class is structured with adults, but with kids a structured class plan can never be followed because of how the kids are feeling, and their attitude. The bottom line: it's got to be fun and unstructured. Go with the flow.

You have the disciplined kids, the attention-seeking kids, the energetic ones, the kids who do not want to participate, and the groaning kids. How do you cater for them all in the one class? With careful thought.

With kids, forced situations don't have happy outcomes, and the same principle applies in a yoga class. Leave them alone. They will join in when they are ready. What about the attention seekers and the groaners? Listen to them, but do not focus on them, and be aware of their needs. Sometimes you might get loners and shy ones; put them in charge, give them responsibility and you will see a change. Regularly, change the postures and the breathing to make it interesting and challenging. Also, throw in some games to make it different, or even some step exercises to Michael Jackson!

Children are usually full of energy and they find it hard to be quiet and restful. Usually with a yoga class, quiet time and centering helps the mood. I have found that this does not work with energetic kids as they need to get rid of that energy to be able to focus. Running, hopping and other strenuous races help to reduce this energy. Any cardio exercise will help this and if they run out of breath, get them to cross hands and tuck their closed fists in their armpits. This will help the breath to return to normal.

Some kids do not like taking their shoes off. That's fine in certain poses. Explain to the kids that in some poses they need to take their shoes off, or they may hurt themselves. Give them that option.

All classes need to be fun. Don't be too regimented about perfecting a pose as long as the child knows the basic posture and its name, and concentrate on the fun side. However, if they complain of pain in a part of the body while doing a posture, always emphasise not hurting themselves but only doing what feels comfortable.

Try to always incorporate into the lesson the various parts of the body, naming them, in order to familiarise the littlies with terms used.

Breathing techniques are very simple instructions and done in a fun way. For example, Kapalabati (skull breath) can be done as a "bunny breath", where the hands are cupped above the ears, upward, and with the inhalation and exhalation opening and closing those bunny ears. More of these examples are described in the next chapter.

Children find it difficult and uncomfortable to breathe through the nose only. Take little steps with them and they will learn gradually.

Different ages in the same class can be challenging. If there are a lot of kids, have shorter sessions for the younger ones.

With the younger ones I use different words to engage them, mainly simplified and colourful words, and I make the games and focusing/meditative segment simpler. Sometimes the older children (primary school) quite enjoy the younger ones' class. A lot of noises captivate them, for example, the cobra/snake hissing, the cat meowing, and the lion growling, to name a few.

Kids with special needs are so lovable as you create a bond to initiate and guide them without tension. Fill the class with love and enjoyment, they get more involved and this activates their nervous system. Take small steps. Visualisation is the key. What works well are:
- A series of integrated yoga postures to strengthen, balance, and increase body awareness.
- Breathing and relaxation techniques to improve concentration.
- Last but not least a well-planned program to bring happiness and wellbeing through gentle, fun and therapeutic yoga.

Use a chair initially with special kids and work from there. This is helpful because of their often weaker strength and balance. They are all kids at heart and they love games and repeating words.

A fun game is to roll the kids in a yoga mat, rolling them across the floor for a distance. Make it a race game, and get another kid to run ahead. This exercise is fun and at the same time, beneficial for the child, as the child's limbs are in a straight position, and with the rolling, the whole body is being massaged.

With all kids, always get feedback at the end of the class. Ask them what they liked and disliked, and this

will help you as a teacher to prepare for the next class.
I have also had instances at adults' and kids' classes, where only one student is present. I never turn them away. I believe he/she made the attempt to come for the class, and as a teacher, I need to respect that.

I had an instance where only one student turned up for class, we both went to a nearby park and did our yoga. The student was so pleased and grateful. This is "Yoga Fit"! Watch hiring agreements. With my hiring agreement of the hall, if I didn't use it I didn't have to pay the hire charges.

Fun Breathing Exercises for Children

Kapalabati/Bunny Breath

- take both hands
- close fingers with thumb inside
- place both hands above head
- breathe in through nose and open fingers
- breathe out and close fingers
  (This is a gentle breath.)

Full Yoga Breath

Imagine one of your hands is a duck.
- support that hand at the elbow with the other hand
- bring all fingers together
- quack like a duck
- bring the duck's beak to your mouth
- hold your lips
- breathe in and out of nose to the count of 1, 2, 3
- extend the count further, if comfortable

Lollipop lady breathing

- take one hand in line with shoulder
- bend elbow
- imagine being a lollipop school person
- stand straight
- close fingers
- school kids are about to cross
- inhale to count of five while opening one finger at a time
- exhale to count of five while closing one finger at a time

Breathing in and out of a straw helps them to understand and control the breath through their mouth. They will then understand the same breathing principle with the nose.

Alternate Nostril Breathing

- imagine there is a little dim light in one nose
- close one nostril
- breathe in and out of the open nostril
- every time you breathe in, the light gets brighter and it fills your nostril
- do the same for the other nostril

When they have mastered this single breathing technique they can use both nostrils, opening and closing each nostril in turn. Remember to emphasise that when they breathe in the light gets bright, and when they breathe out, it gets dimmer.

Dragon Breath/Bhastrika

- sitting on heels
- hands on knees
- breathing in and out of tummy
- while exhaling, pump the air out vigorously as if squashing a balloon
- close hands to form fists
- move hands up and down, round and about, in tune with the breath (dragon moving)
- on each exhalation open the fingers and move

Ujayi Breath/Psychic breath/Darth Vader breath

This is a focusing breath. Opening mouth and breathing in and out of the mouth, as if trying to put out a birthday candle. Then closing mouth and still breathing the same way.

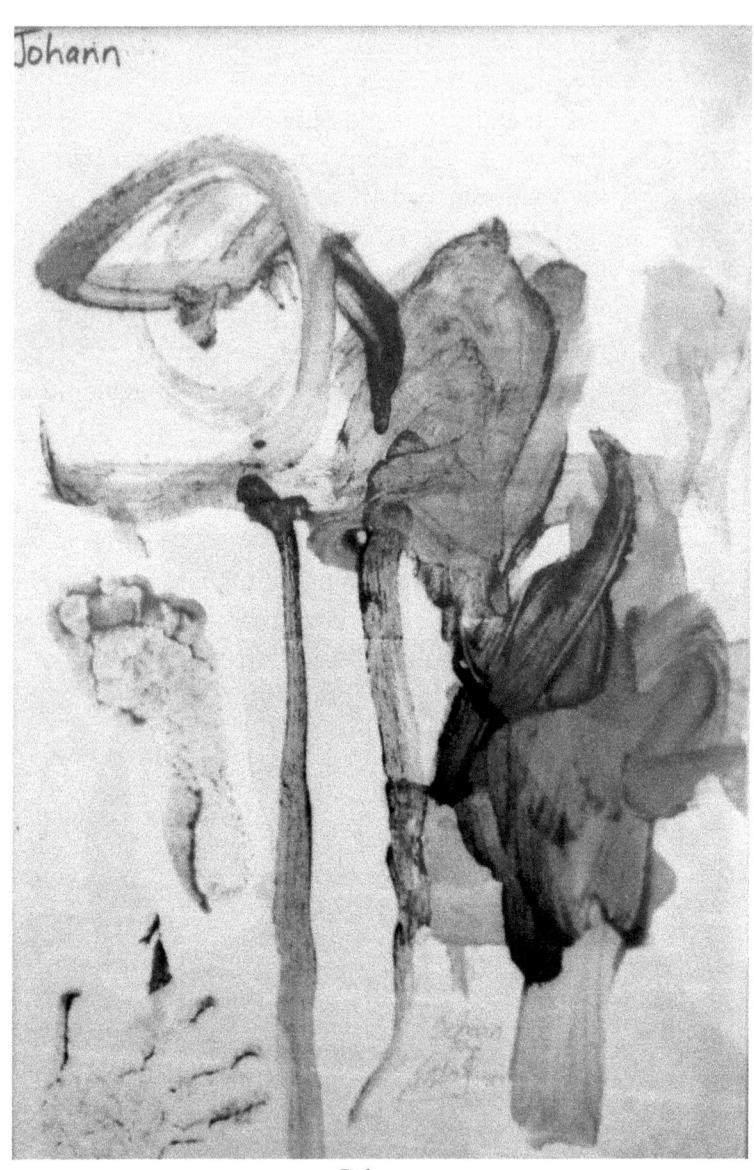

Johann

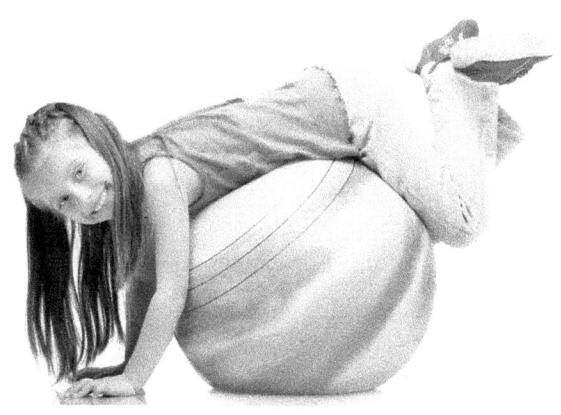

Games for Kids

This is definitely a hit with the kids. I always throw in a game or two, depending on the class and the numbers, always giving firm instructions with a trial run. Balancing games work well with children who are not focused and listening. Breathing games also help them with awareness of how we should breathe. Take into consideration the ages of the children, both in individual and team games, to be fair. There might be one or two kids who will refuse to take part because of an injury. Assess the situation and give them referee duty or supervisor duty and this works wonders. They might be hard on some others for vengeance! So be aware.

If the weather is good, take the kids outdoors into the fresh air to do some of the games. Beware of the ants and remember the shoes-and-hat policy! Kids love races. This can be in the form of running, hopping on one leg, skipping, frog race and duck race, to name a few. Relays also make a difference as they are a team effort. Watch the bigger kids as they may tend to be cliquey and the littlies are disadvantaged.

Here are some of the games:

Ducky Ducky Quack Quack

- all children sitting/standing in a circle
- blindfold a child
- blindfolded child walks around the circle to music (touching the backs of the chairs, or if the other kids are standing or sitting on floor, another child should guide)
- when the music stops, the blindfolded child will gently touch the child and say, "Ducky ducky"
- the touched child will reply "Quack, quack"

The aim of the game is for the blindfolded child to identify the voice and name the other child. Not too much touching in this game.

Pass the Parcel

Pass a cushion or stuffed animal to music and the person who has it when the music stops, picks a card, and does what the card says (usually relates to doing a posture, a breathing technique or something funny).

Sticker – eye game (eye exercise)

Give the kids a coloured sticker to put on their nose. Do eye exercises and they guess the colour of the sticker.

Straws and ping pong ball (good breathing exercise)

- four rows of children
- two teams, and each team facing each other
- kids on their chests
- a straw and ball are given to the child at the start of the row
- this child will blow the ball through the straw to the child opposite until the ball reaches the last team member

A windy day or a fan is a bit of a challenge

Car/truck driving competition (good tummy exercise)

- four rows of children
- two teams, and each team facing each other quite a good distance away
- kids seated straight with legs extended (if insufficient room, the kids other than the first kid can have their legs spread out in a V)
- a round object will serve as a steering wheel
- the aim of the game is to hold the steering wheel in front of chest, and at the same time, move one leg at a time towards the opposite partner and hand over to the partner to take over

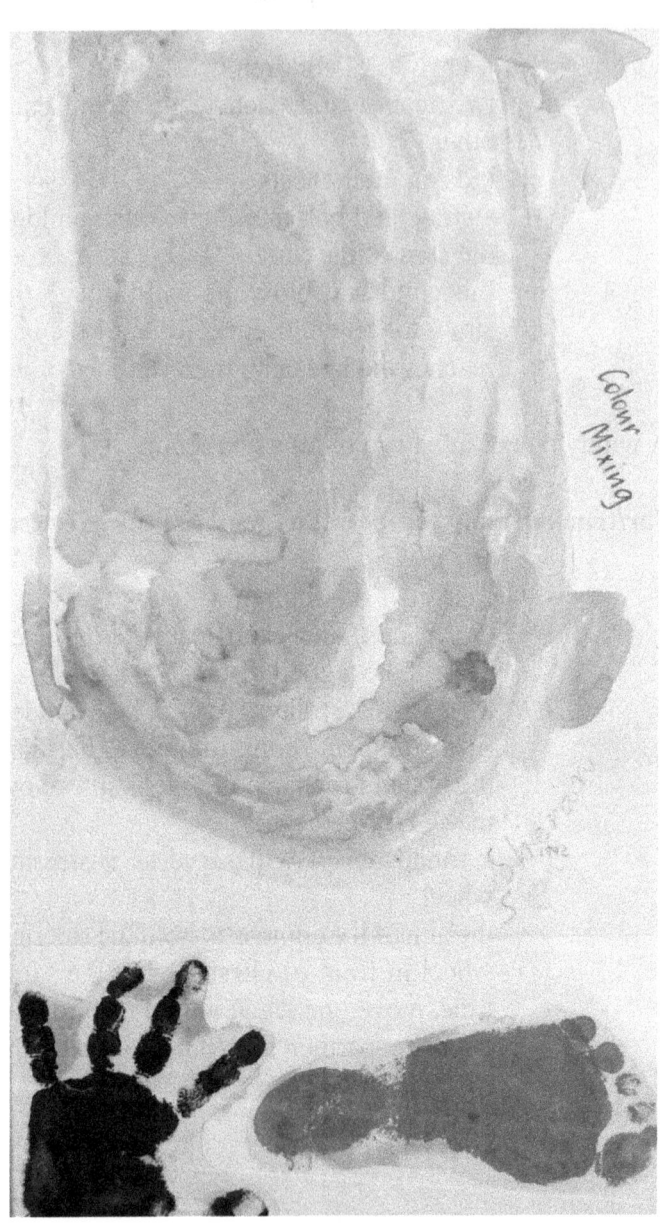

Sheran

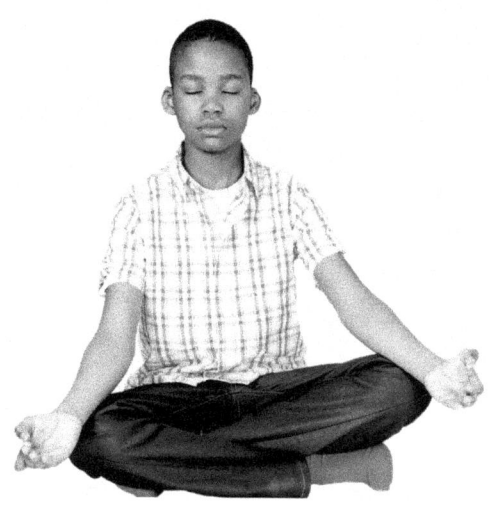

Relaxation for Kids

Kids love this segment. Just before quiet time a quietening/relaxing breath will help. The moment I turn the lights off and switch on the music the kids zoom into another world and it is so beautiful to watch them.

Some kids can be restless during relaxation. I get these kids to roll onto their sides or onto their tummies. Others like crossing their legs. As long as they are comfortable. The same with their hand positions.

Conscious relaxation

Touch your head, breathe in, now breathe out and relax your head…
Touch your face, breathe in, breathe out and relax your face…
Touch your neck…
Touch your upper chest…

Touch your chest…
Touch your tummy…
Touch your hips…
Touch the top of your legs, breathe in, breathe out and relax both your legs…
Both your hands by your side and completely relax your whole body and … let go. Your body is sinking, sinking into that big soft, soft cushion and you feel so light…

Older kids

Fold both your fists, tense your hands, breathe in, tense, tense, now let go.
Keep doing this with each part of the body. If you feel they are still not relaxed, try the conscious relaxation above.

I also read out a visual journey or imaginary adventure, giving them choices of colours or shapes, for example, a kite. When they come out of the relaxation, I am able to then have a talk on their chosen colours and shapes etc, and their imagination has no limit. This helps with their expression, and also their language skills.

There are so many benefits in a simple five to ten minute relaxation session achieved simply by turning off the lights, lying in a comfortable position and putting on some soothing or nature music. The kids just switch off to another zone. Many teachers have commented on kids' better behaviour after relaxation. Even if there is no yoga class/relaxation, the kids will ask for some soothing music to "chill out". This is how we are all meant to be, we should all take some time out.

What are Alpha Brain Wave patterns?

Alpha, Beta, Theta and Delta are different brain waves that function in different ways. High Alpha brain waves indicate a person is in a relaxed but aware state.

Alpha Brain Wave patterns can be stimulated by:

- Relaxation
- Mood
- Place
- Music

All children, whether they are:

- over-active
- sluggish
- special needs
- angry
- over-active
- moody

…will benefit enormously from relaxation.

Our nervous system is divided into two parts, the sympathetic nervous system, often known as the "fight or flight" or "red switch", and the parasympathetic nervous system which I refer to as the "tune in and chill out" or "blue space". They are two completely different responses, and in our daily life we do experience both states, that is, the "red switch" and the "blue space". The "red switch" uses much of our energy, and the "blue space" reloads our energy. By being in the "red switch" position, we deplete our energy, and this results in stress-related illnesses, such as behavioural problems, insomnia, fatigue, digestive and respiratory disorders, and even coronary problems. It also affects our immune system. In a nutshell, if we are constantly in the "red switch" position we are cranky, difficult to get along with, plus have health problems and generally are not living a happy, healthy, or peaceful life.

By familiarising kids with the basic tools of relaxation, and being in the "blue space":

- It calms the kids' behaviour and emotions, thereby minimising inappropriate behaviour.
- Kids' actions are calm and peaceful.
- Their studies improve, they are placid, and find it easier to get on with both their peers and teachers.
- They have a caring attitude, and generally are more grounded, in tune with one another and listen more attentively.

Meditation/focusing is a challenge, short spans can be beneficial. For the younger kids, display various shapes, colours or toys, and get them to lie on their chest with hands on their chins, observing the various items. Cover the items and challenge them to remember what they saw, for example, the colours, shapes etc.

Older kids enjoy the above activity as well, but if you wish to try a more challenging activity for them try puzzles or games to find the missing letter etc.

As a team, both the younger and older ones can visualise a candle flame and watch the flame, what colours surround it, how many flames etc. This activity of meditation/focusing helps restless kids, and, generally, the cognitive brain function is used. Concentration, memory and general studies are improved.

An example of one of the imaginative journeys that I have taken the children through:

- Firstly, I ask them a few questions on the various parts of the body, pointing them out (especially if there are little kids).
- I show them the different colours of the rainbow.
- We do a conscious relaxation of the body, where every part of the body is alternately tensed and relaxed, or place the hands on each part of the body, breathing in and tensing and while breathing out and letting go of that part of the body.
- Allow the body to then "sink" into the floor beneath.
- With closed eyes, imagine and visualise sinking into a big, big cushion while your body feels so light.
- Now imagine yourself as a tiny, tiny person going into your heart. Your heart is full of happiness and love. See a rainbow over your heart, with all the beautiful colours: red, blue, yellow, green, purple, violet and indigo. Choose a colour, and imagine this colour flowing through your body. Imagine you are wrapping ribbons of that same colour of love and peace all around you (relaxing for five to ten minutes).
- Move your hands and feet and bring your knees onto your chest, holding them

firmly and moving them from side to side like a beetle.
- Coming onto your side, gently come up into a seated position. Keep both your palms at your chest and keep your eyes closed.
- "May you take the happiness and love that you felt in your heart and body to everything in this world. Have a great day or week and peace go with you."
- Have a discussion time to keep them in the "blue space" zone, and to improve their communication with each other. For example, who had a red ribbon? Did your ribbon fit all around you?

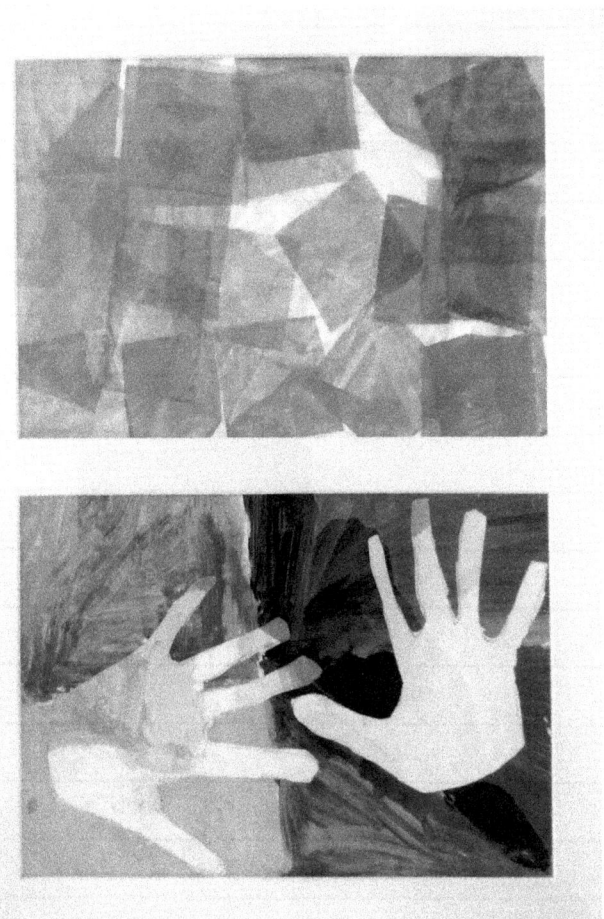

Jivan

Notes

PART 5

YOGA DICTIONARY

Yogi/yogini	male/female who does yoga
Satyananda	system of yoga developed by Swami Satyananda
Iyengar	system of yoga developed by BKS Iyengar
Jivatman	soul
Paramatman	universe
Om Shanthi	peace to the universe
Asanas	postures
Mandala	circular symbol
Om	sacred triple sound
Yama	avoidance
Niyama	observance
Prana	force/energy
Pratyahara	withdrawal of senses inwardly
Dharanaya	concentration
Dhyana	meditation
Samadhi	bliss
Hatha	physical
Raja	mental control

Pranayama	breath
Pran	oxygen
Ayama	extend/control
Tattwas	elements
Chakra	energy centre/wheel
Muladhara	force centre at base of spine
Swadisthana	sexual centre
Manipura	force centre at solar plexus
Anahata	force centre at cardiac plexus
Vishuddhi	plexus in the pharyngeal region
Ajna	force centre or trigger point between eyebrows
Sahasrara	thousand petal lotus/crown centre
Poorak	inhalation
Kumbhak	retention
Rechaka	exhalation
Nadi Sodhana	alternate nostril breathing
Tadasana	mountain
Sitali	cooling breath
Kapalabati	skull/bunny breath
Bhastrika	dragon breath
Ujayi	psychic breath

REFLECTION

> "I have not failed. I've just found 10,000 ways that won't work"
> Thomas Edison

As I come to the end of this book, please take the time to read, enjoy and practise. Take small steps to reach the summit of love and peace, experiencing both pleasure and pain along your journey.

As you meditate or come out of a relaxation, make simple positive affirmations over and over. If you don't feel comfortable with this, make a recording which you can use often.

Suggest the word "peace", and ask the kids to make an affirmation based on this. For example, "I send peace to all the world".

Affirmations

- I will climb all hills today slowly and mindfully.
- I will today **b**reathe, **e**at, **s**mile and **t**alk with love.
- I will listen today to my heart.
- I am grateful for today.
- I enjoy my work/studies. I shine in everything I do.
- I always have wealth, physically and emotionally.
- All my barriers are small. I meet them with loving thoughts.
- My life is filled with love and peace.
- I will today look for positives; turning all negatives into positives.

BUT WITH LOVE

Fly like a bird
With love and laughter;
Not with impatience
Not with anger;
Not with intolerance,
But with love.
The past is gone,
The future out of grasp;
Be in the now,
But with love.

Final Thought

I wish to extend gratitude to my family, friends, work colleagues, associates, teachers, students, and all whose paths I have crossed in my life.

In appreciation, the 'But With Love' poem is for you all. Thank you! Please take time to read it and send it on.

I have dedicated a section in my book and website to breast cancer and multiple sclerosis wellbeing. I will make a donation from this adventure of telling my story and sharing it with others, to aid these two organisations.

For more information about The Power of Yoga, Adriana Silva, YogaDo Classes and much more visit
www.yogado.com.au

Notes

Notes

www.ingramcontent.com/pod-product-compliance
Lightning Source LLC
Chambersburg PA
CBHW051702090426
42736CB00013B/2498